Sometimes My Socks are in the Freezer.

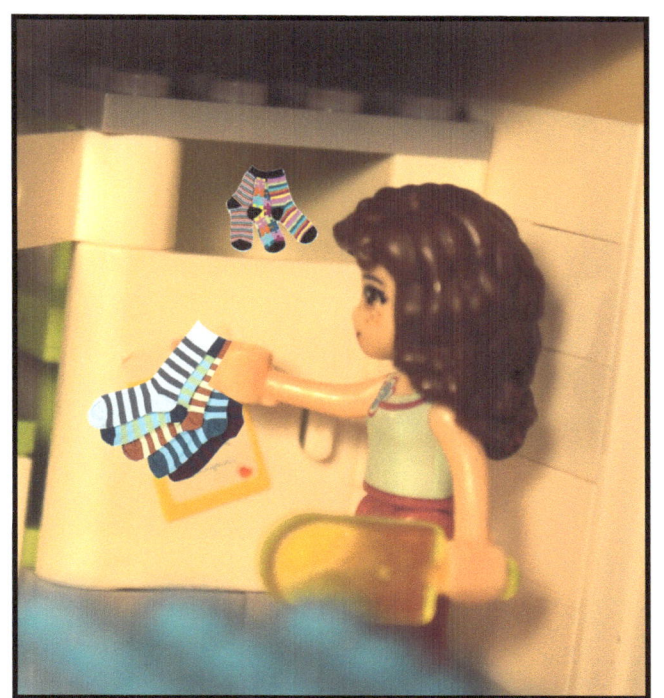

A Book About Narcolepsy and Automatic Behavior

To my daughter Zoey,
I love you to the moon and back

To my husband David,
Thank you for always believing in me

Sometimes My Socks are in the Freezer

A Book About Narcolepsy and Automatic Behaviour

Amanda Stock

astock204@gmail.com

ISBN-13: 978-1516854431

ISBN-10: 1516854438

First Edition 2015

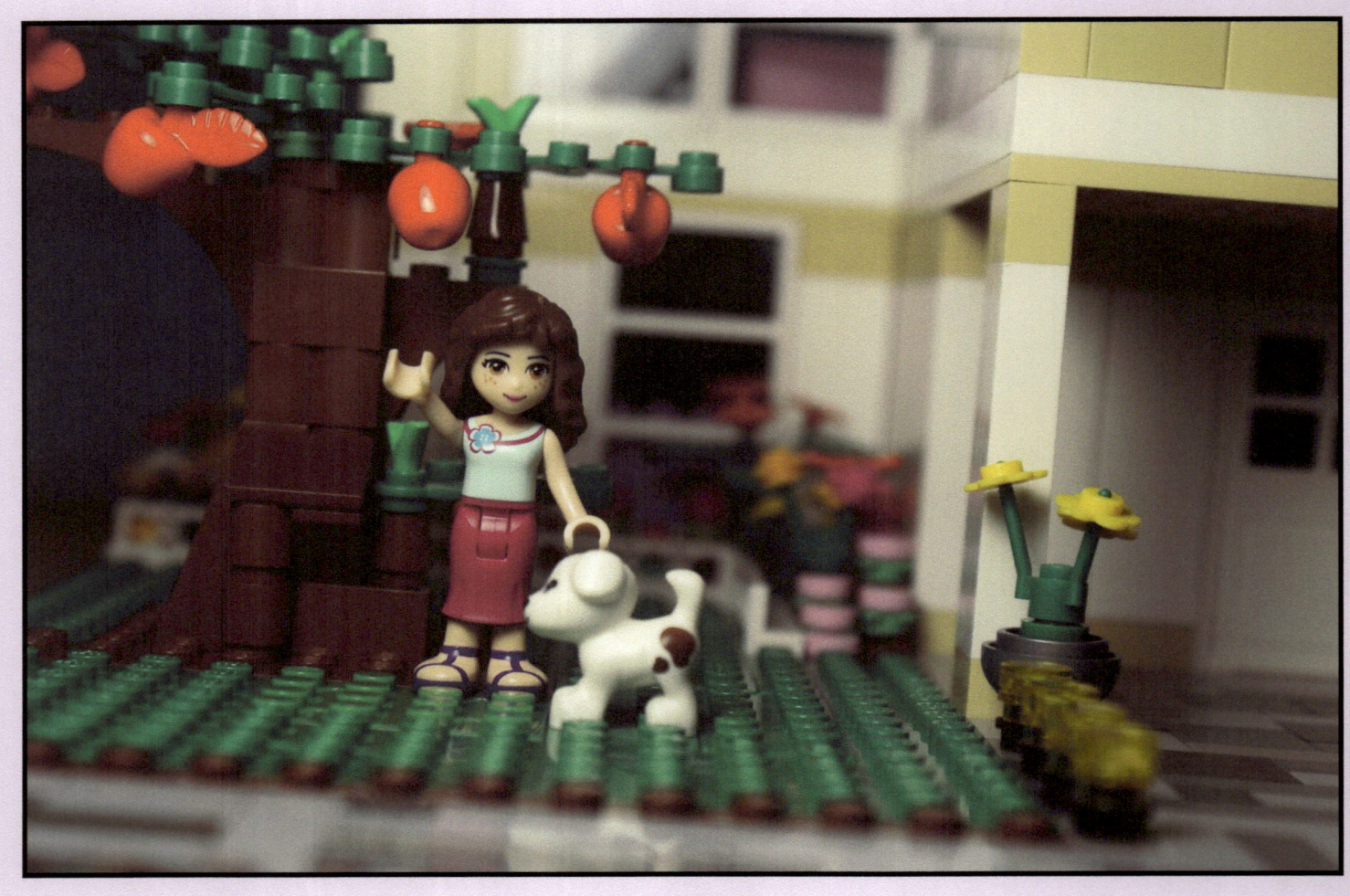

Hi! My name is Zoey.

Sometimes I find my socks in the freezer. You may think that's silly but for me it's pretty normal. My mommy has a sleep disorder called Narcolepsy.

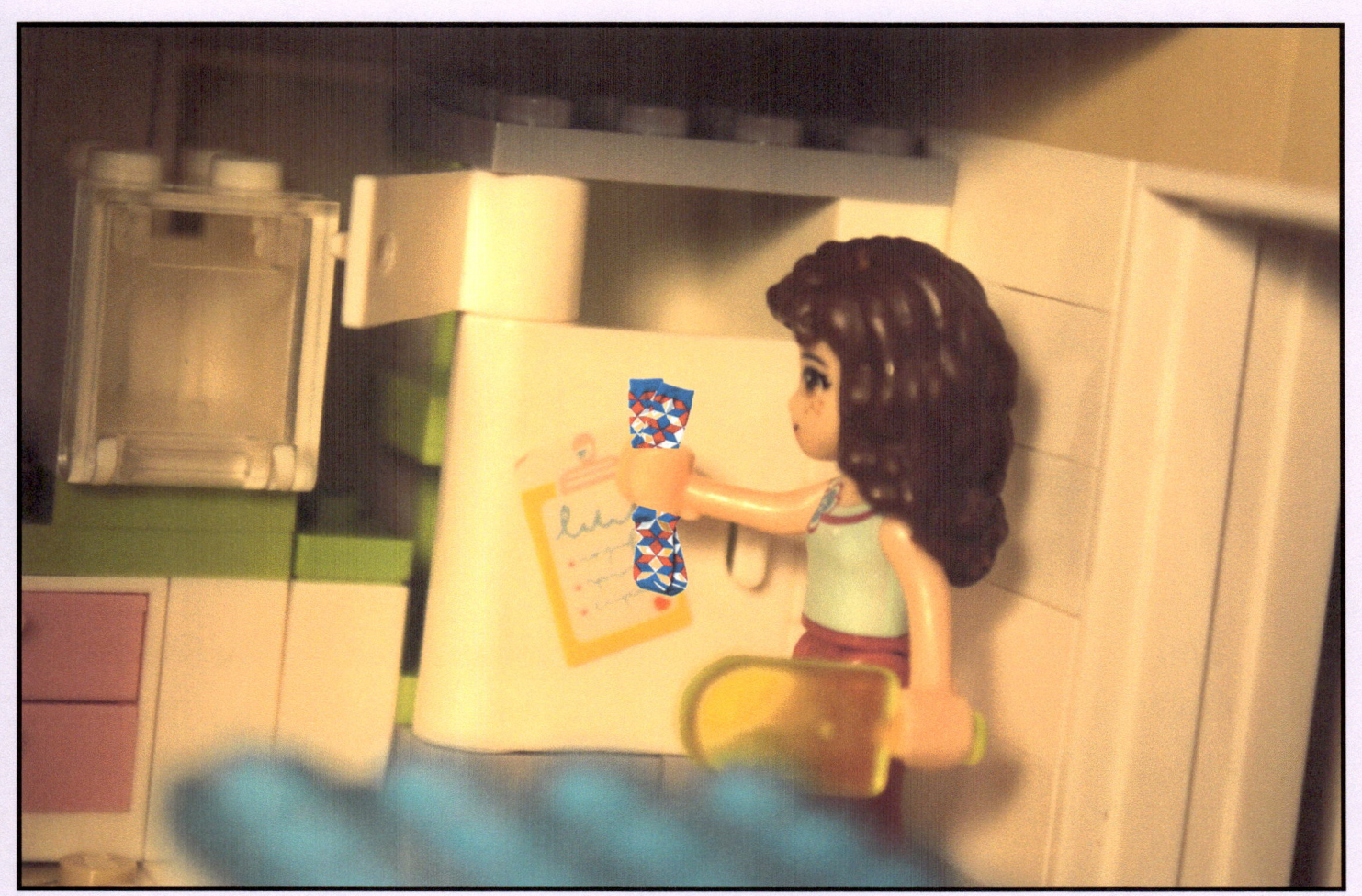

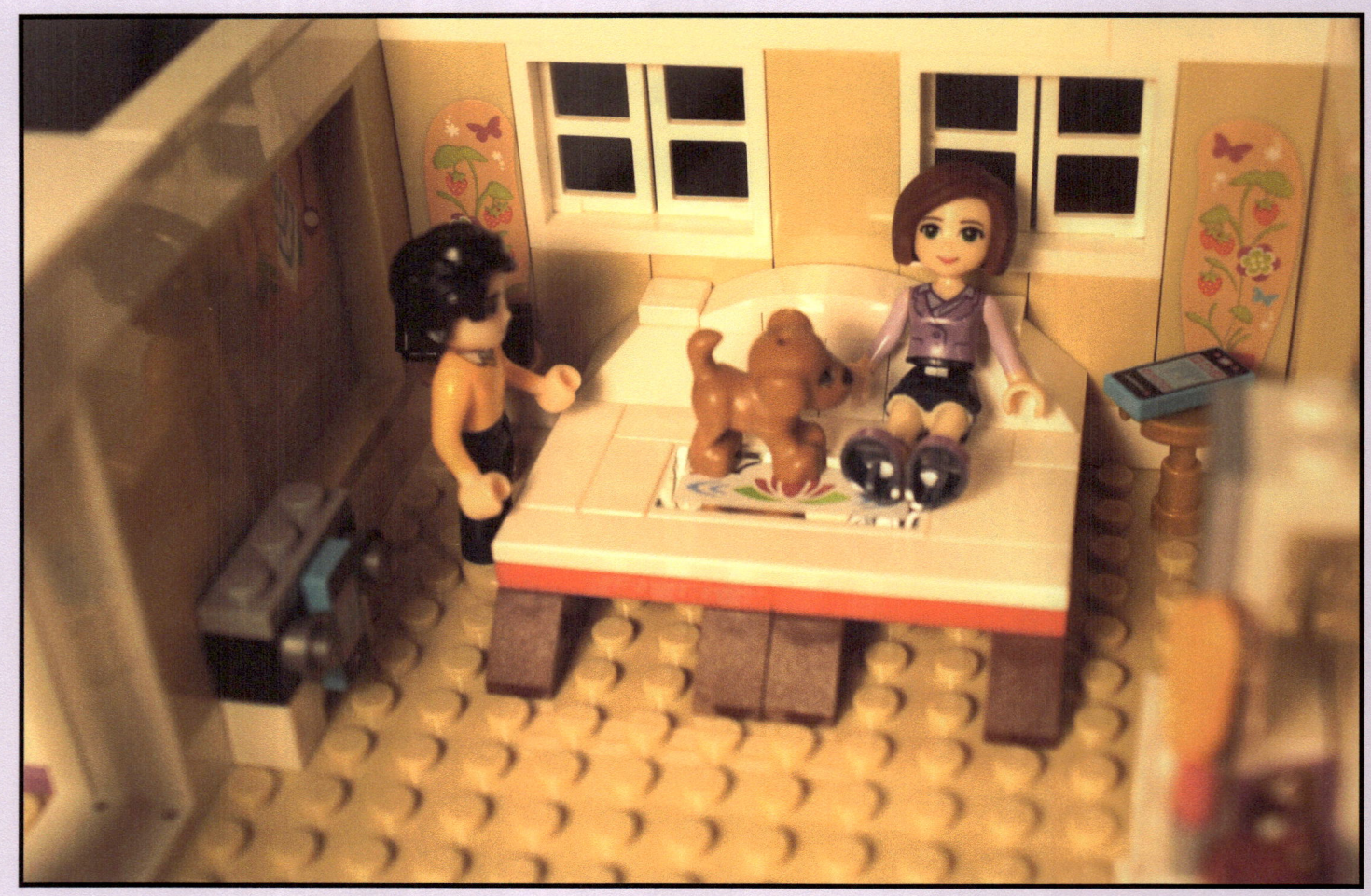

When someone has a sleep disorder it means their brain works differently. Narcolepsy makes some people tired all the time. My mommy loves to sleep in on weekends but daddy wakes her up because it's not good for her. Getting extra sleep doesn't help but napping does.

Narcolepsy not only makes mommy feel sleepy it also makes her fall asleep when she doesn't want to. Sometimes even though mommy is awake part of her brain thinks it's sleepy and falls asleep. This is called Automatic Behavior. When that happens mommy doesn't remember anything. This is when she does funny stuff and I find my socks in the freezer.

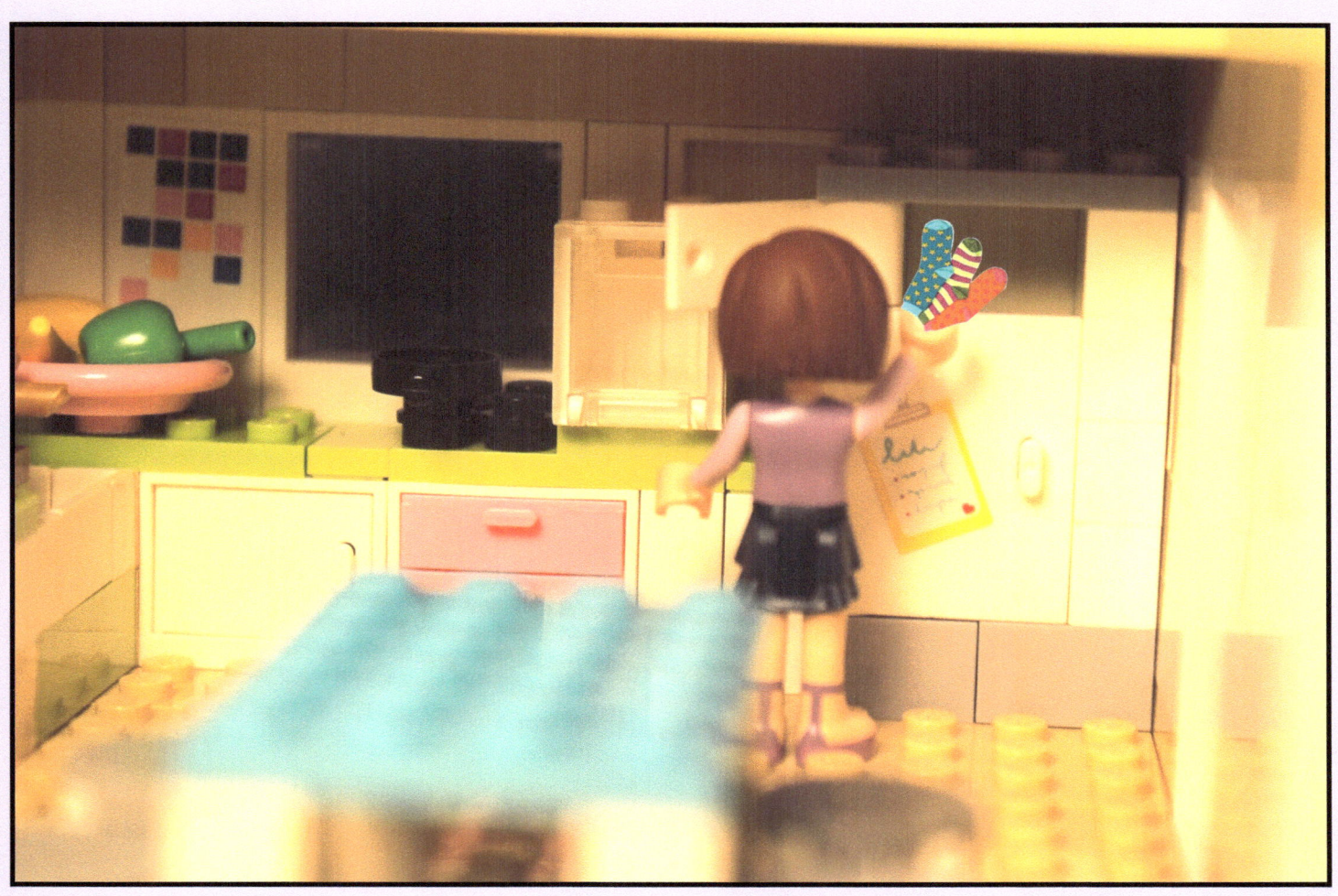

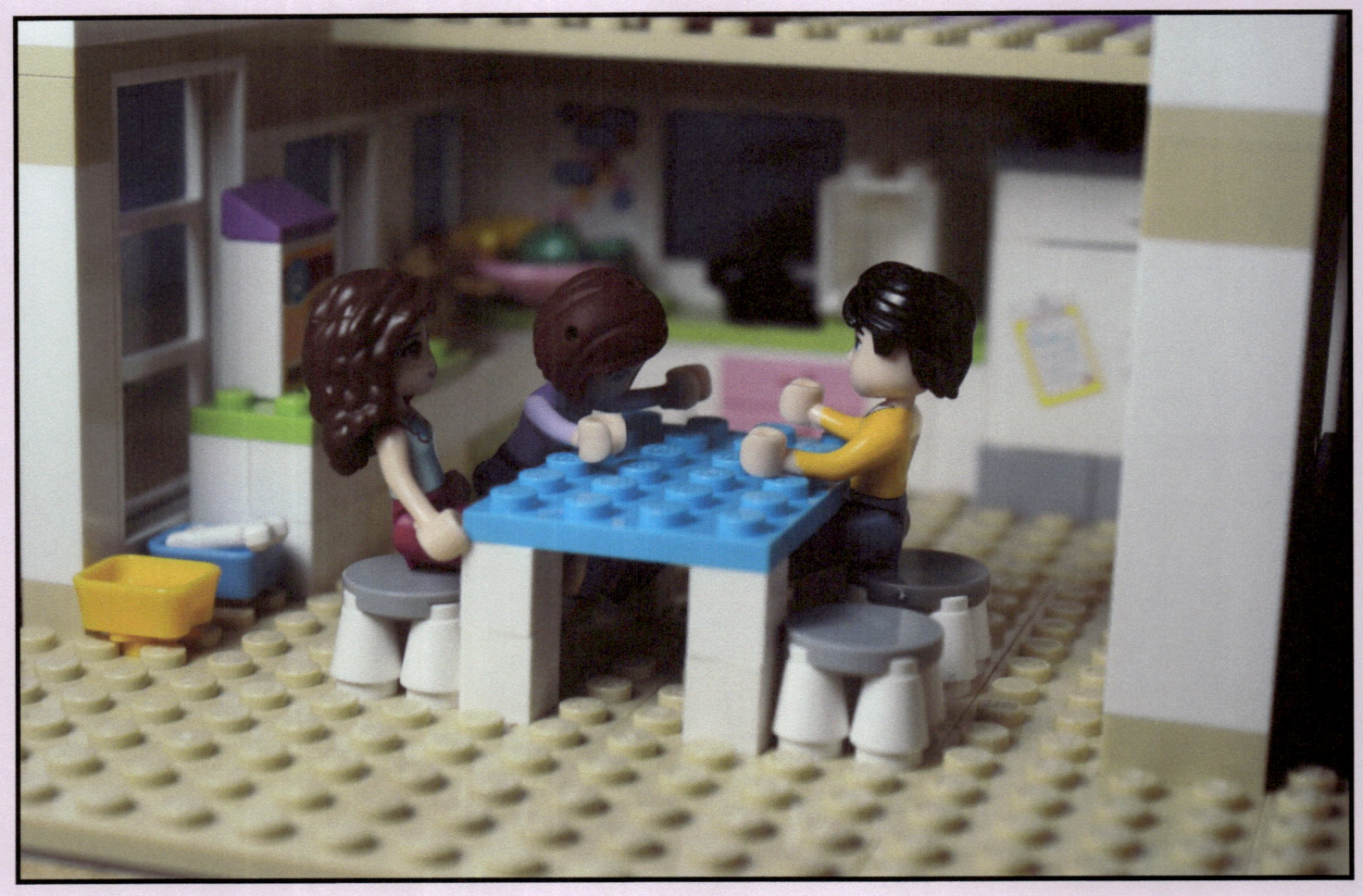

Mommy repeats herself a lot because she doesn't remember what she told me and will keep telling me until she remembers. One time she was trying to tell us stories from when she went to summer camp and she kept forgetting words. She was really upset.

It is important for our family to stay very organized so important things do not get lost. My mommy keeps a calendar of our important events and has special spots for keys and papers.

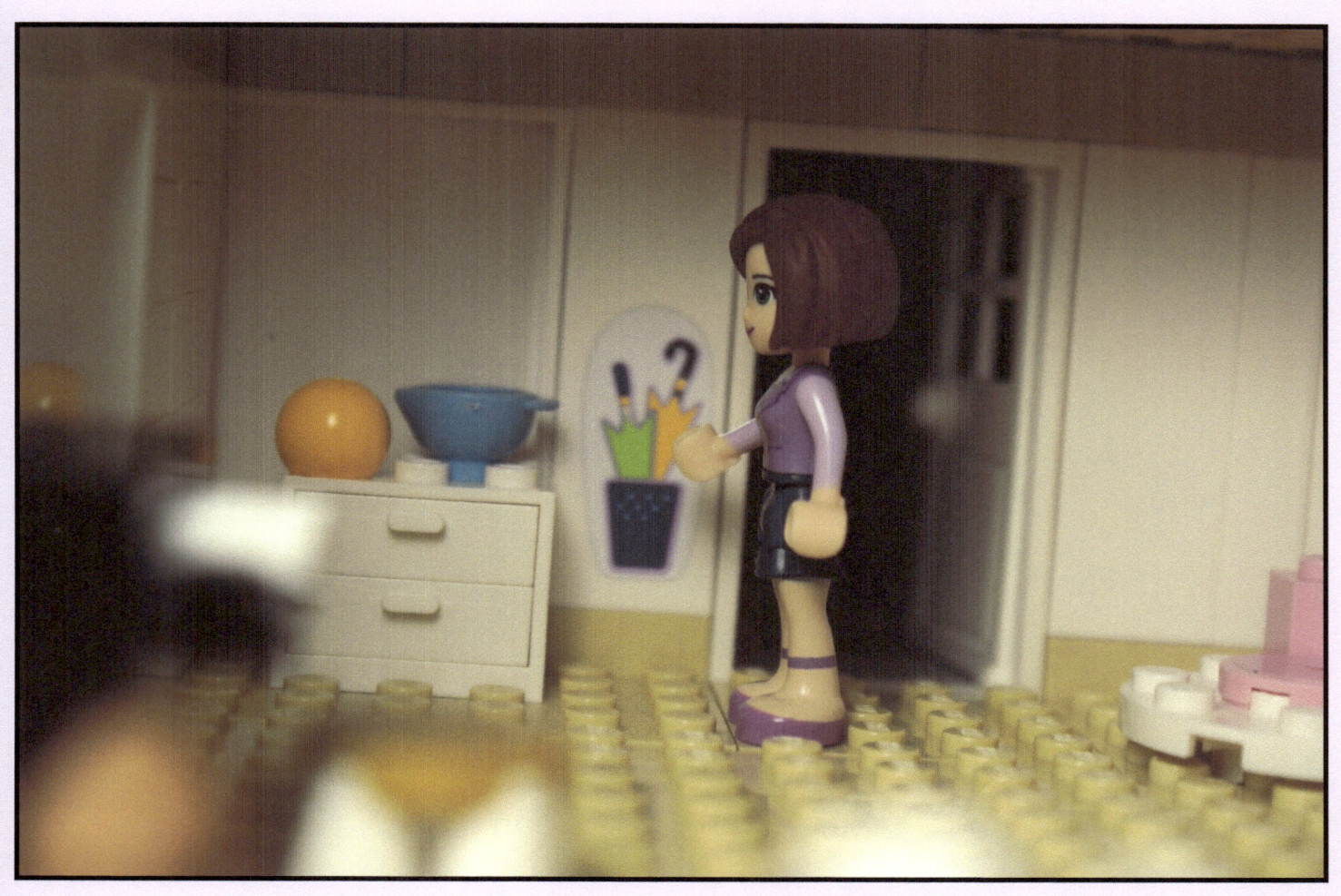

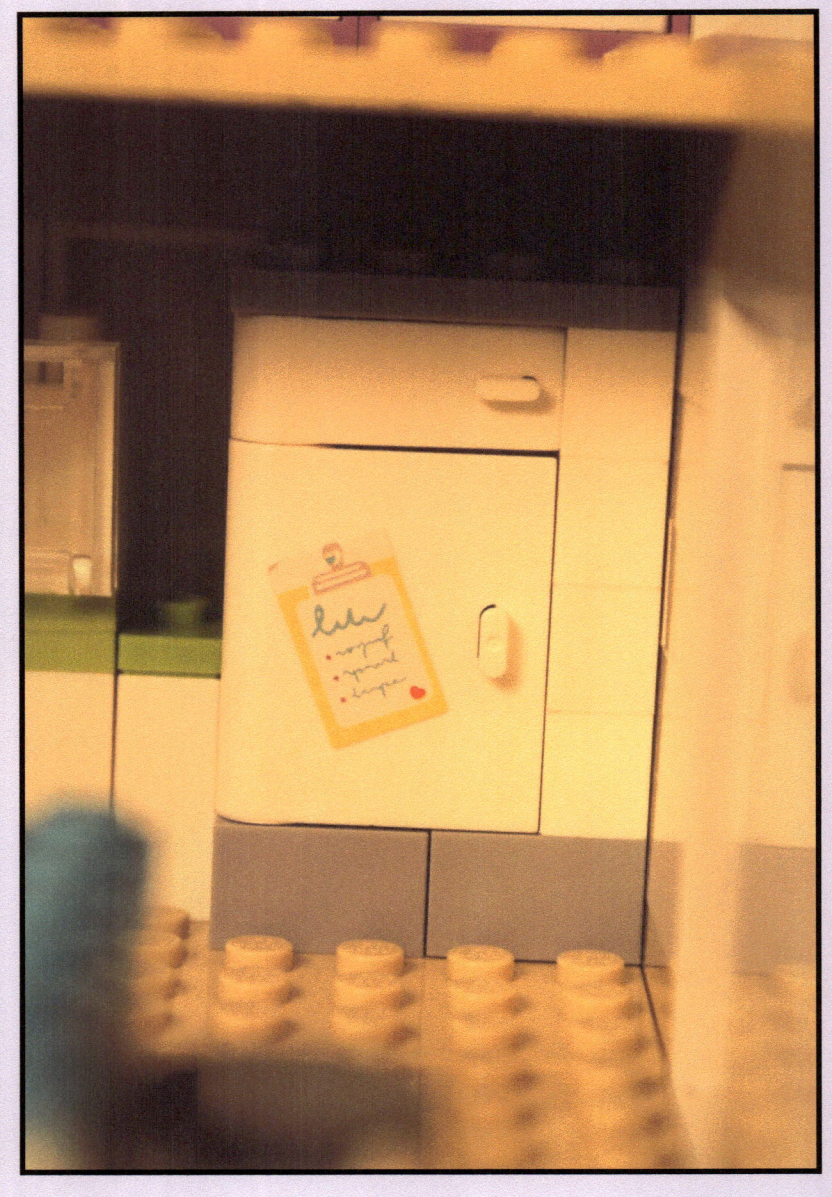

We also have a "to do" list on the fridge so we all can work as a team to keep the house clean.

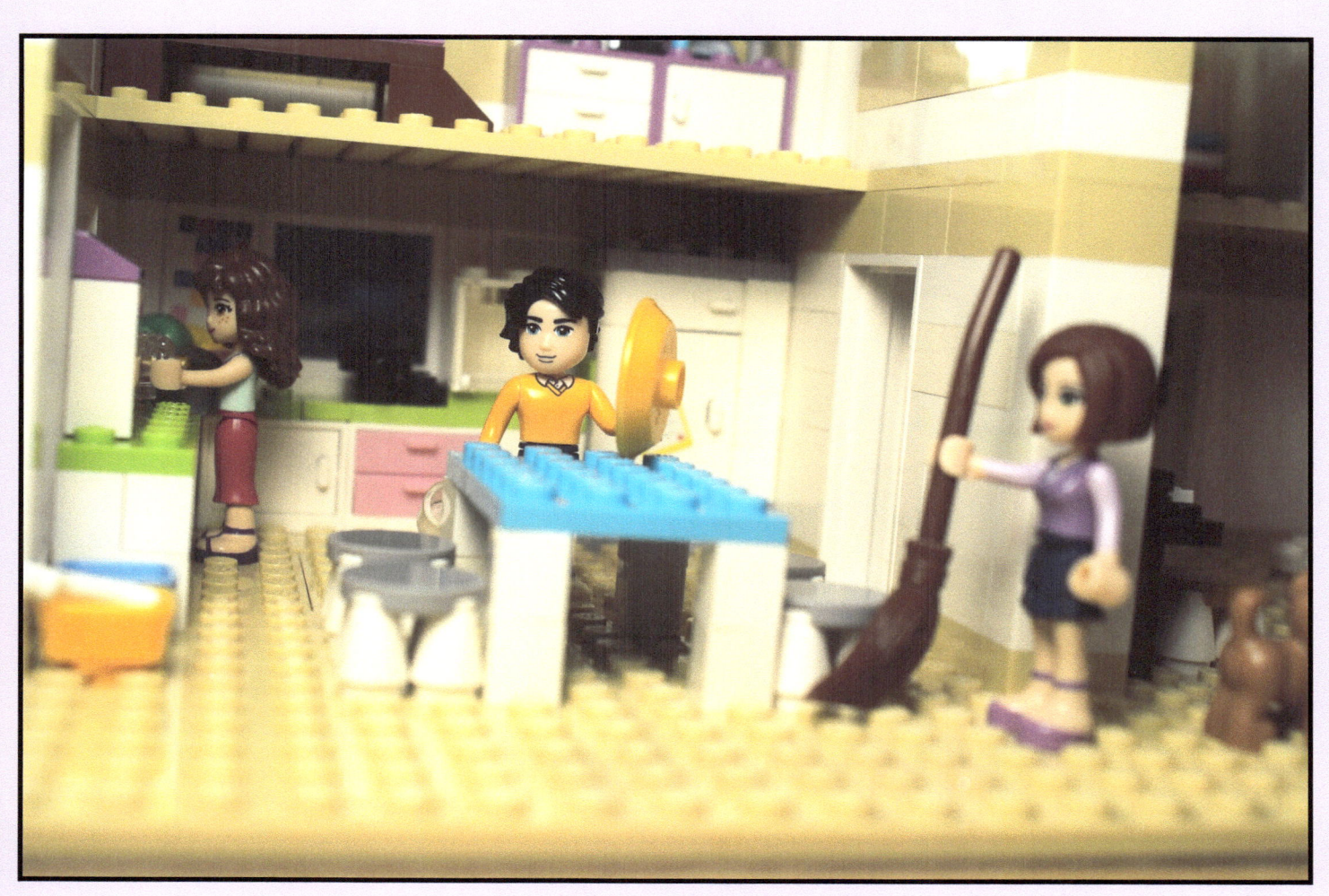

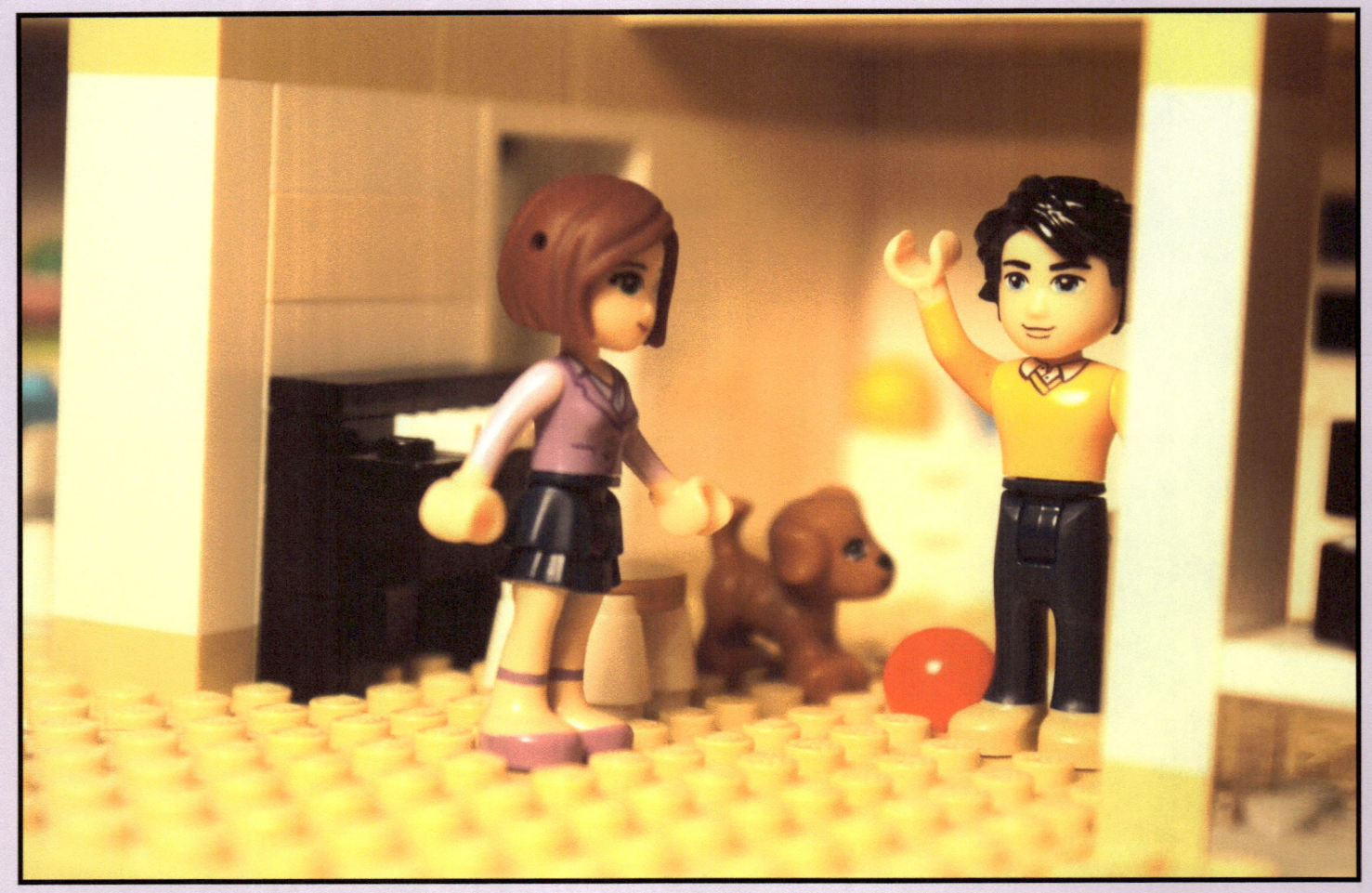

Sometimes daddy has to tell mommy to take a nap when she has had a stressful day at work. He says that stress makes mommy's symptoms worse so it is very important that she takes naps during the day when she needs them.

It was scary for my mommy when she was younger and did not know what was wrong. But now that she does she makes sure to follow the doctor's orders so she can be the best mommy she can be!

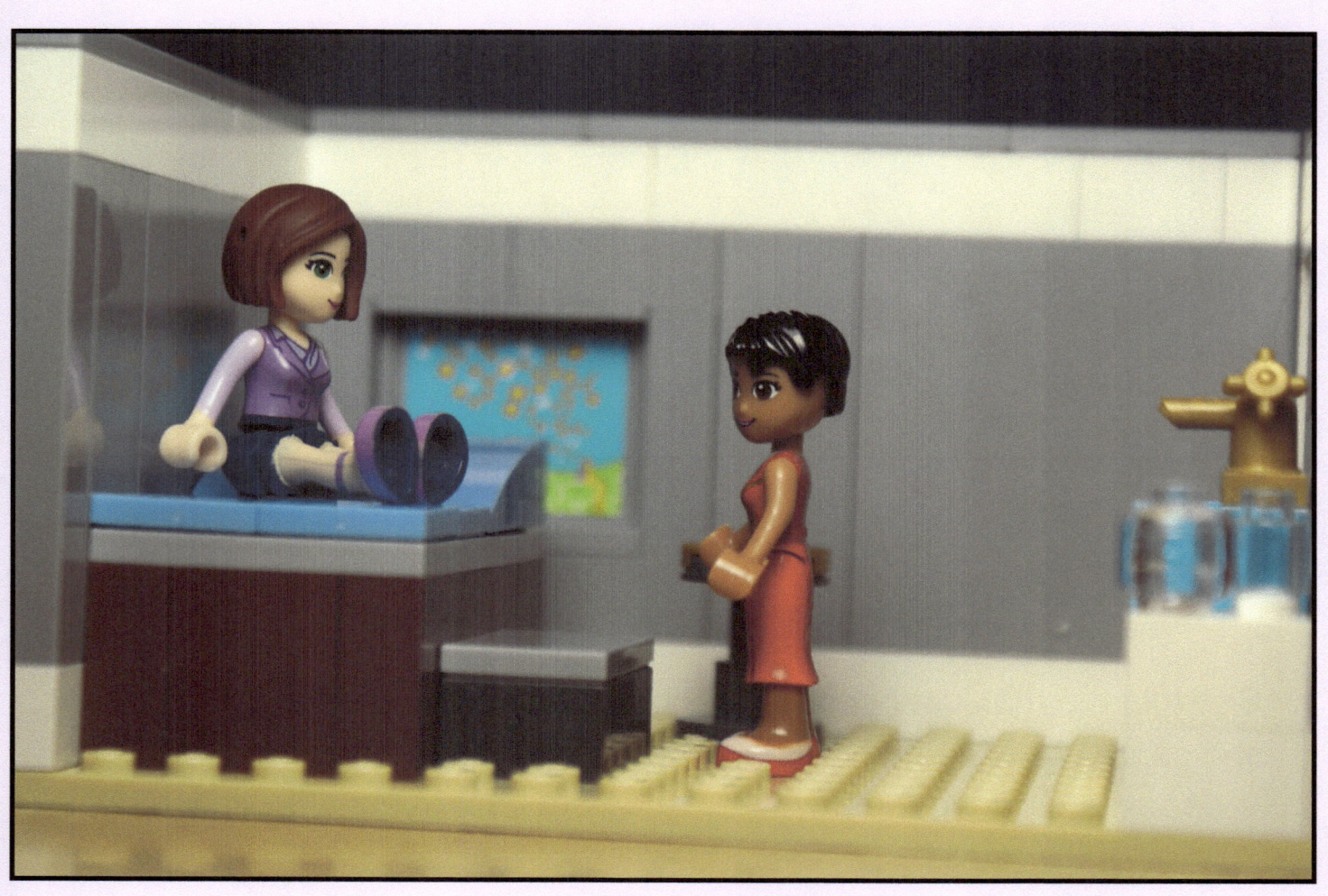

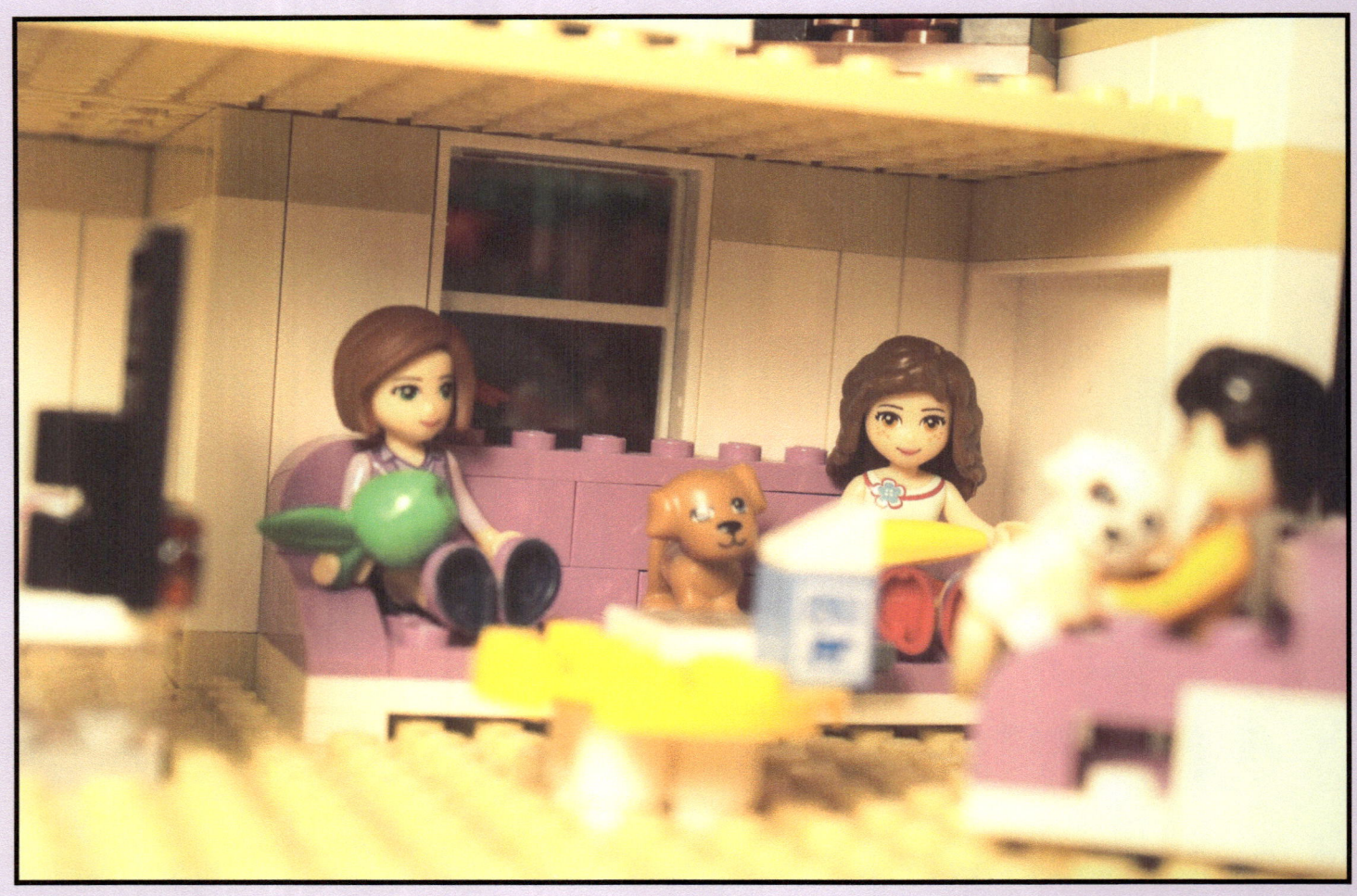

She told me that just because she has a sleep disorder does not mean she cannot be a normal mommy! She takes special medication to keep her awake during the day and we try out best to eat a healthy diet.

When mommy is feeling really good she goes for a bike ride with the dogs or takes me for a walk to the park. She even has a bed time. Keeping a regular bed time helps her feel better.

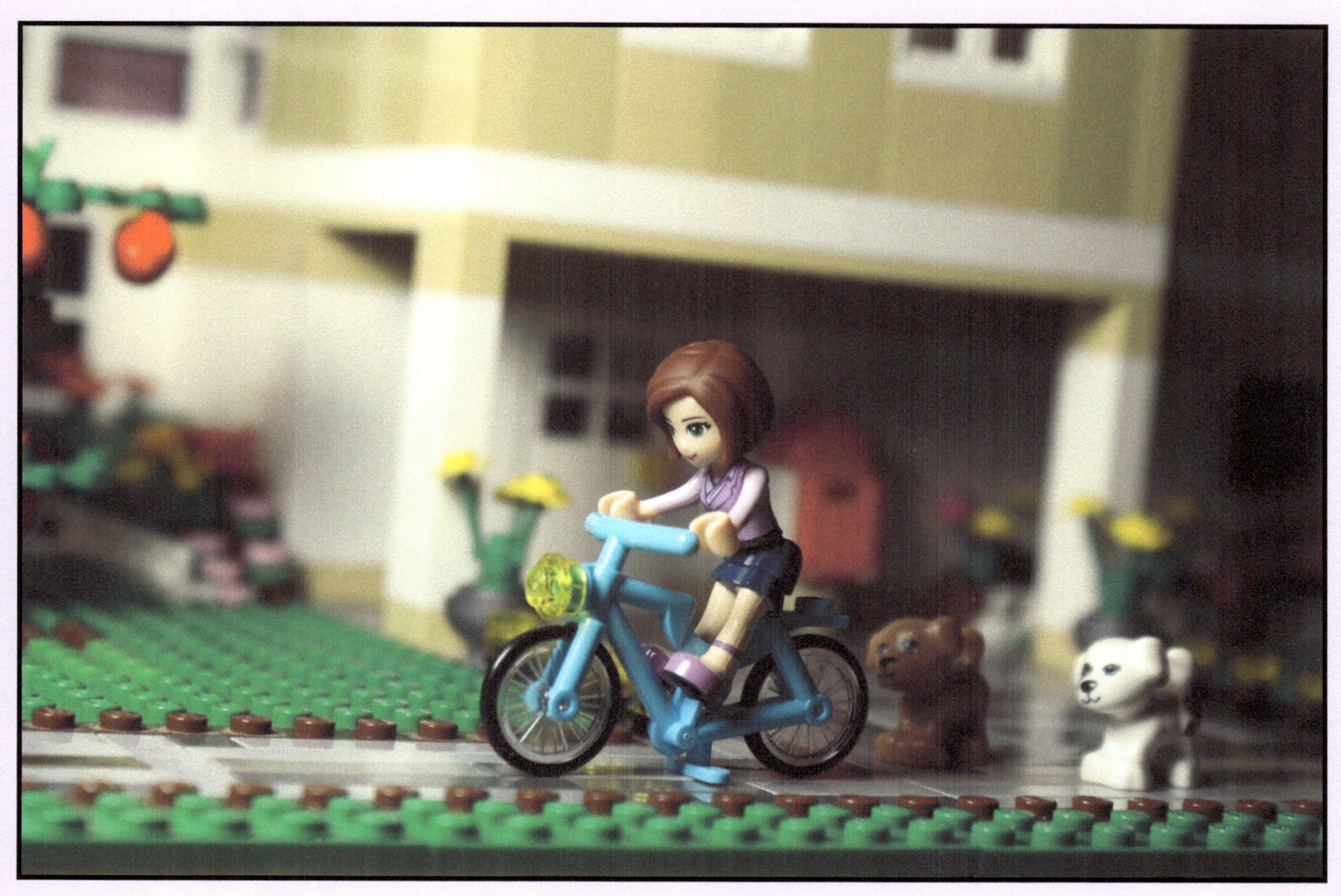

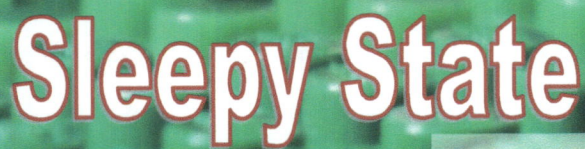

Sleepy State

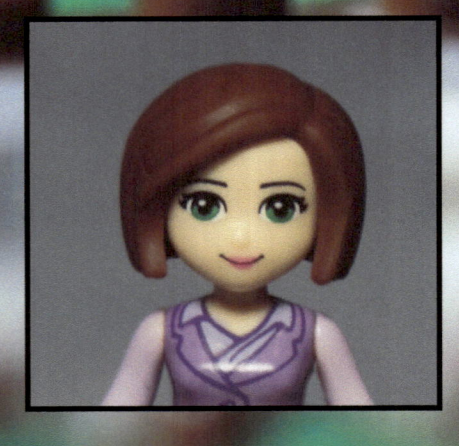

Non-Driver Identification Card

ID #: 1234567890

Tired, Jill
123 Main Street
Springfield, Sleepy State 10203

DOB: 08-12-1980   Sex: F
Issue: 08-16-1996   Height: 0' 2"
Expire: 08-16-2022   Eyes: Brown

My mommy doesn't drive anymore because of the Automatic Behavior. She did when she was younger but she always tried to get a ride when she could. When the doctor told her she had Narcolepsy she gave her license up.

A lot of people with Narcolepsy can drive but mommy's Automatic Behavior scares her and she is too afraid of what might happen. Daddy said he will teach me how to drive when I'm older and mommy will cheer me on from the backseat.

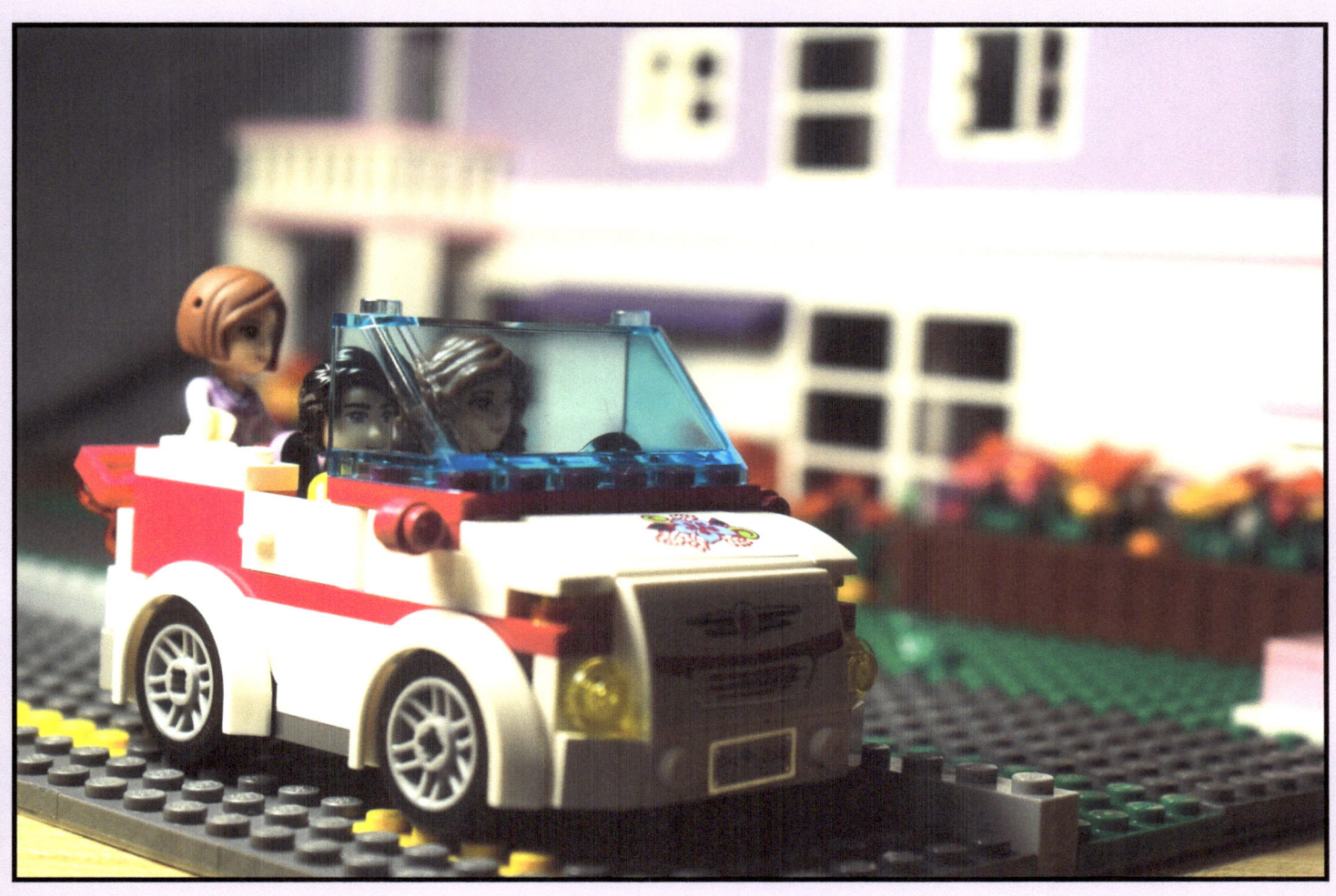

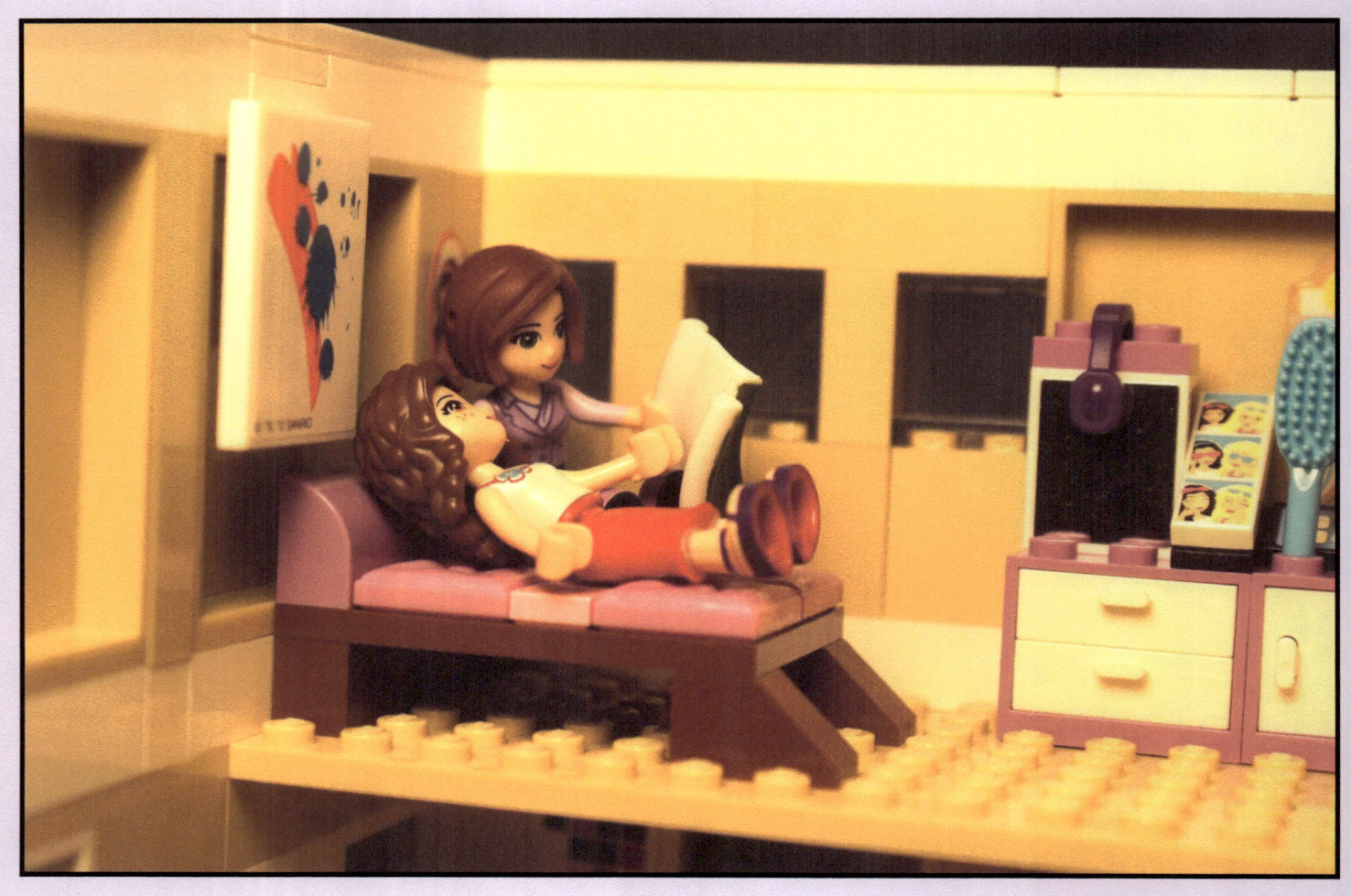

My mommy may have Narcolepsy but she is still pretty great!

Even when she puts my socks in the freezer.

Follow up questions

- What was your favorite part of the book?
- Did the book remind you of _____?

  Person in your life with Narcolepsy

- What things in the book reminded you of _____?

  Person in your life with Narcolepsy

- Does anything in the book bother you?
- Is there anything else you would like to learn about Narcolepsy and Automatic Behavior

Definitions

- Sleep Disorder: When a person's sleep patterns are different then they should be
- Narcolepsy: When the brain goes sleep during times the person should be awake
- Automatic Behavior: When the brain or it's parts fall asleep while the rest of the body is still awake
- Symptom: When a person does something "weird" or different that lets them or others know they might be sick.

Books in the Talking to Kids About Narcolepsy Series

Book 1 - Automatic Behavior: Sometimes My Socks are in the Freezer
Book 2 - Excessive Daytime Sleepiness: My Dad Naps Too!

Coming Soon!

Book 3 - Cataplexy
Book 4 - Sleep Paralysis
Book 5 - Hypnagogic Hallucinations

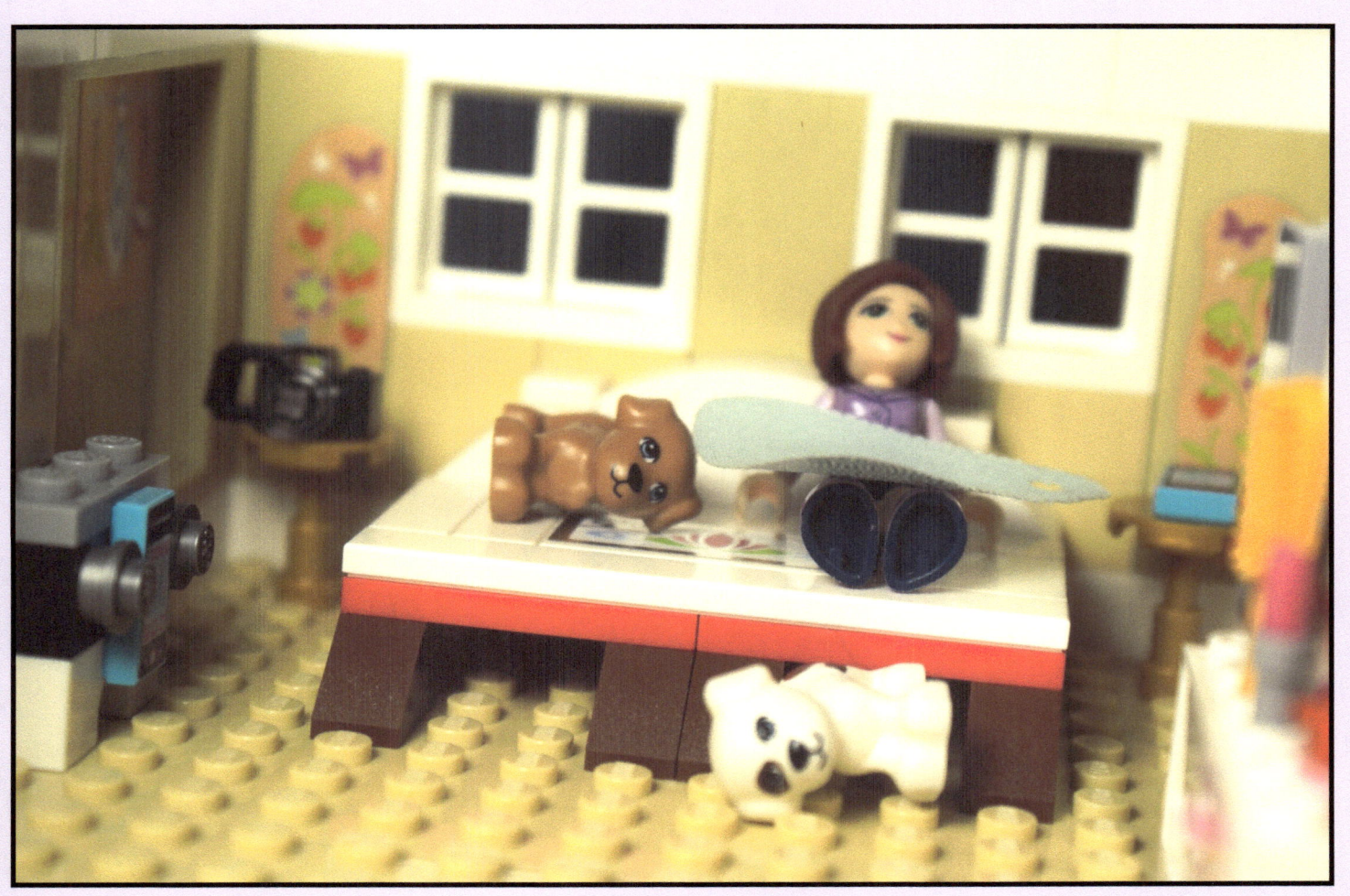

About the Author

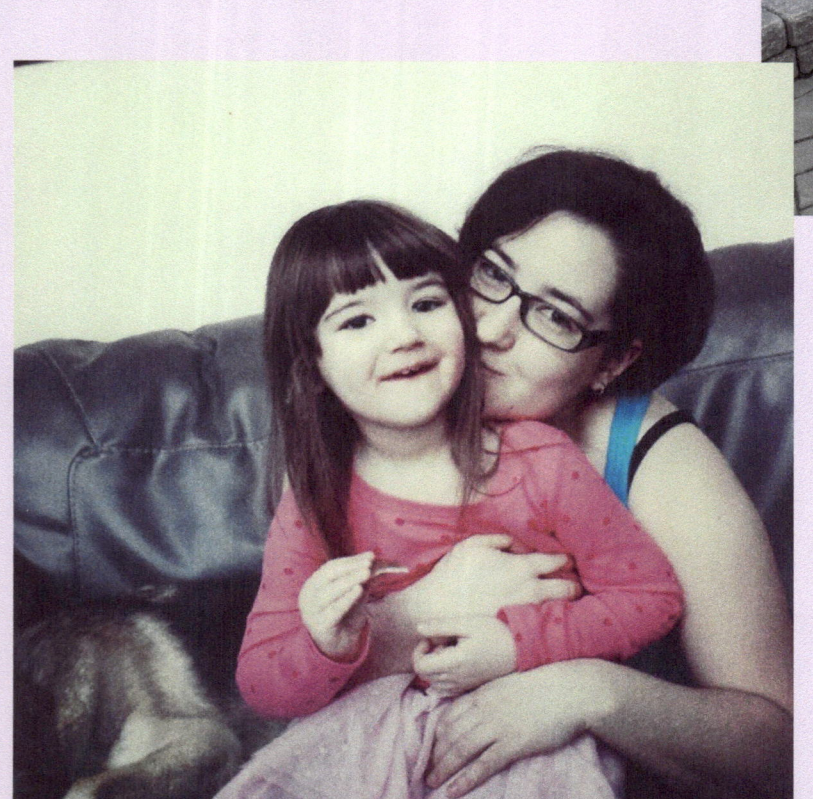

Amanda Stock is the author and photographer of My Dad Naps Too! and the upcoming books in the Talking to Kids about Narcolepsy series. These books were written to assist adults with explaining what Narcolepsy is to a young child or other people in their life. Having a young daughter, Amanda knew this would be an obstacle she would one day face and set out to find a solution.

Amanda is a wife and mother living with Narcolepsy. Like most Narcoleptics she began showing symptoms at age 15 but was not diagnosed unto age 26. Receiving that diagnosis was a huge relief. Understanding what the problem was and how to manage it has made a big difference in her life.

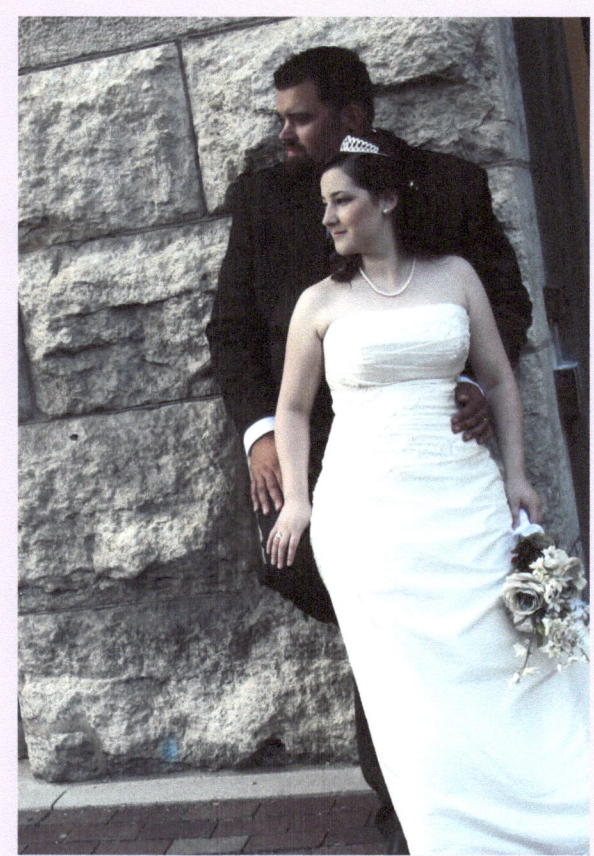

The Talking to Kids about Narcolepsy book series has been a three year project due to the author's incredible lack of drawing skills. This book series is in no way authorized, sponsored, or endorsed by The LEGO Company but could not have completed without their amazing product.